Clean Eating

The Amazing Way to Eat Healthy and Lose Weight

** Includes 25 recipes **

Avoid Processed Food and Reset Your Body's Natural Balance

By

K.A. DeWolf

Introduction

The difference between your food's natural state and what winds up on your plate is getting bigger every day. Manufacturers are adding high fructose corn syrup to everything from spaghetti sauce and bread to roasted nuts and yogurt. Artificial preservatives are present in almost everything, whether canned or not. Conventionally grown vegetables are sprayed with harsh, harmful pesticides. Livestock are treated with hormones to force unnatural growth, and large amounts of antibiotics to counteract the maladies that arise from factory farming conditions. All of this ends up on your plate.

With the rise of these practices, the world has seen skyrocketing rates of obesity and cancer. According to Livestrong, obesity rates have risen 214% from their levels in 1950. Colon cancer is up 60% in the same timeframe, heavily linked to an increase in red meat consumption. The cost of this is enormous-- not only to the sufferers of these diseases, but also to taxpayers.

Lax regulation and corporate lobbying have enabled companies to bypass common sense restrictions, using unquestionably harmful chemicals on, in, and around your food.

In this book, I'm going to present you with an alternative. I'll show you how to improve your health, lose weight, and eat sensibly. By the time you're finished reading, you'll have all the tools required to make the easy, infinitely beneficial transition to real clean eating.

In Chapter 1, "What is Clean Eating?", I'll be defining clean eating as it's presented in this book, and highlighting the difference between minimally processed and conventionally processed food.

The second chapter, "Stocking Your Kitchen", will give you information about the essentials to keep in your home, from fruits and vegetables to pantry staples and spices. I'll give you tips on healthy oils and alternatives to things you might buy now. I'll show you how to bring your plate to life, enhancing and augmenting the natural deliciousness of fruits, vegetables, and meat.

Chapter 3, "Health Benefits", will break down the immediate health benefits of transitioning to a clean diet. There, I'll be presenting the nutritional differences between conventional products and their clean alternatives.

In Chapter 4, "Sourcing Your Ingredients", you'll be shown the process of finding whole ingredients. From the farmer's market to the grocery store, with a little diligence you can find and purchase whole, even home-grown fruits and vegetables.

Chapter 5, my favorite chapter, is "25 Delicious Recipes for Every Meal" I'm going to share some of my favorite recipes with you. Enjoy!

K.A. DeWolf

Table of Contents

The trademarks that are used are without any consent, and the publication of the trademark is without permission or backing by the trademark owner. All trademarks and brands within this book are for clarifying purposes only and are the owned by the owners themselves, not affiliated with this document.

Chapter 1: What is Clean Eating?

To define what clean eating is, it might be helpful to first define what clean eating is not. It's not a fad diet. It's not a diet at all, really. Unlike the innumerable wild guesses at what "works" for the highest number of people, clean eating is an age-old practice.

For modern people, it's an essential lifestyle change, and a fundamental shift in the way you see your food. It's a return to a time in which you didn't have to worry about how many harmful, synthetic pesticides were on your fruit. A time in which high fructose corn syrup in a loaf of bread would seem patently ridiculous. Before you had to fret over whether or not your meat was full of antibiotics and artificial growth hormones.

Eating "organic" is distinctly different from clean eating. Organic guidelines are not at all stringent about the amounts of pesticides used-- only their origin. Many demonstrably harmful chemicals, such as the carcinogenic copper sulfate, are used in exorbitant amounts on so-called "industrial organic" farms. In fact, in many cases, the highly specialized fungicides and pesticides developed for conventional factory farming are less toxic than those from natural sources. If you've ever cracked the spine on a biology textbook, you know that plant-derived toxins can be incredibly virulent and potent.

Clean eating is the practice of knowing the origins of your food. Clean eaters buy from local farmers and ranchers, and know about their raising and growing practices, and it's a lot less trouble than you might think. You'd be hard pressed to call up Tyson Chicken and get a tour of one of their farms; in fact, there are laws preventing exactly that, bought and paid for by the companies themselves. They don't want the consumer to see the origin of their food, because the truth is unquestionably ugly.

It's important to remember, however, that not all companies have questionable practices or harmful ingredients. Most of your staples, especially grains, can be easily and ethically sourced, and their ingredients and preparation audited.

My advice is to eat local and seasonal whenever possible. Meat should be sourced from local butchers, fruits and vegetables from nearby farms (whether directly or at farmers' markets), and grains from local companies if any exist. This is commonly referred to as "locavore" eating-- that is, eating food with origins within 100 miles of your home (distances vary between proponents). You'll find that much of your food can be gotten for far less money in this way, since the added costs of transport, storage, retail markup, advertisement, and corporate profits aren't attached to the final price.

The essential tenet of clean eating is knowing where your food comes from. What better way to retain control over your own food than to grow it yourself? Many plants are incredibly easy to grow in minimal space. Tomato plants and squash are especially popular, but you should always check with your state's growing authority to find out what grows most effectively in your area. There are innumerable resources available to would-be growers online, as well. Growing your own food from heirloom seeds can be incredibly fulfilling, and depending on what you grow, you can preserve and can (or dry) your food to be eaten in times when the plant does not produce.

"Backyard chickens" are a great source of eggs, and meat if your population is large enough. Keeping chickens is easy, and inexpensive in the long term when compared to buying the same amount of eggs you'll receive. If you can't process the chickens you've raised yourself, a local butcher would likely provide the service for a small fee. This practice has been gaining traction recently, especially with people in rural and semi-rural areas.

Now that you know just what clean eating is, and have been given a handful of potential implementations, I'd like to go more in depth and talk about the absolute essentials for every clean eater's kitchen.

Chapter 2: Stocking Your Kitchen

In my opinion, the trick to clean eating comes down to making cooking and eating your own food as appealing as possible. Therefore, my first suggestion is this-- learn to cook. You can go through a lot of trial and error, but the recipes at the end of this book should set you on the path if you aren't there already.

It's impossible to cook great meals without a well stocked kitchen, though. Your refrigerator, pantry, and spice cabinet should be the first three places you think of when you want food; not restaurants, fast food joints, or boxed dinners. I have a list of the absolute necessities from each category for clean eating and great cooking. The first and most important place to stock is your refrigerator (or counter, in some cases).

20 Essentials

1. Tomato

I cannot overstate the importance of keeping a few tomatoes around, though no more than you can eat within a few days since you should buy them fully ripe. They're best eaten at room temperature, but despite assertions to the contrary, storing them in the refrigerator does nothing to degrade their taste or texture. From sauces to sandwiches, chilis to calzones, their uses are seemingly unlimited.

2. Corn

The humble, abundant, and well loved ear of corn is a lot more versatile than people give it credit for. It's not just a boil and butter affair. If you soak a whole ear of corn in water for a half hour and bake at 350-400 degrees for about as long, husk and all, you'll find it incredibly sweet and refreshing. After this treatment, the husk is infinitely easier to remove, as well. It can even be eaten raw, and kids especially enjoy it that way!

3. Zucchini

My favorite squash is zucchini, for a lot of different reasons. It's incredibly versatile, it tastes fantastic, and it's great for you. When prepared, a whole pound of zucchini is only 82 calories, but it provides a full quarter of your daily fiber, half your Vitamin A RDA, and a whole host of other nutritional goodies.

In recent years, many people who follow a low carb or raw food diet have begun spiralizing zucchini to make veggie noodles, and I can attest to their deliciousness, especially in salads. Personally, I prefer them sliced thin and baked with a dusting of spices, but they're fit for far too many dishes to list here. From zucchini bread to chunky chili, you can't go wrong with zucchini.

4. Bell peppers

For me, bell peppers are the ultimate addition to many dishes, and every stage of ripeness has its own unique character and usage.

Green bell peppers are by far the most common and inexpensive. They're the immature stage, and their flavor can be best described as bitter and spicy, though not in the same way as most other "peppers". In my opinion, they're best used in tandem with onions, garlic, and celery for a complete flavor enhancing mix for beans.

Orange bell peppers are fruity, vibrant, and far less bitter than green bell peppers. They can be eaten raw, and are especially good in things like summer wraps along with spinach, tomato, and other fresh vegetables. I find they lose much of their unique flavor when cooked or roasted, and don't perform as well in that role as red bell peppers.

Red bell peppers are the mature stage of the vegetable, and their flavor is rich and complex. The base "bite" of the green variety has subsided along with all bitterness. Instead, they're refreshing and savory, especially when roasted.

5. Onions

Onions are potentially the most useful thing for a well stocked kitchen. They add a depth of flavor and savory character that simply can't be obtained any other way. They can be a real pain to cut, but the rewards are more than worth it.

From beans to stir fries, you can't go wrong with onion. They also caramelize beautifully in a skillet.

6. Spinach

Spinach is absolutely indispensable in my kitchen. Honestly, I shoe-horn spinach in wherever I can in just about every recipe I can. Don't worry, the list at the end of the book isn't spinach-themed or anything. But it's incredibly nutritious, super delicious, and simply can't be beat as filler for wraps and salads.

7. Kale

Kale, until recently, was almost entirely ignored. Pizza Hut used it to decorate their salad bars-- not in the bowls, but in the bed underneath them. We now know that kale is an absolute nutritional powerhouse, and it's really caught on with the health-conscious crowd. It's a wonderful addition to any green smoothie, and I personally can't get enough of it sautéed with a little apple cider vinegar, salt and pepper, and minced garlic.

8. Mushrooms

Mushrooms are an absolute necessity, in my opinion. When simmered in a little oil and spice, they make an incredible sauce of their own that can add a whole new dimension to other dishes.

They're also rich in vitamin D if exposed gills-up to sunlight, a practice more and more companies are adopting.

9. Cauliflower

Cauliflower is a lot more versatile than people think. It can be boiled and ground to make filler for meatballs or hushpuppies, blended to make wonderful alfredo-like sauces, or press-fried in spice.

At the end of the day, cauliflower needs to be treated with care though. If it's not prepared correctly, it's likely to turn you off of it entirely. If this has already happened, grab a nice recipe and give it another chance. You'll be glad you did.

10. Broccoli

The much-maligned broccoli doesn't deserve its rotten reputation, in my opinion. From the time most people are kids, they refuse to eat broccoli, and I can't imagine why! It's nutritious, low-calorie, and incredibly delicious on its own (if prepared correctly) or in dishes.

Even better, when slow-cooked along with vegetable scraps and water, it gives broth an exceptional and unique flavor.

11. Green beans

Fresh green beans are a world away from the limp, gray-olive things you find in cans. They're crisp, light, and intensely flavorful. Like many other vegetables, they're best prepared by steaming to preserve their essential character rather than boiling or frying.

However, even doing those things, fresh green beans make all the difference, whether they're front-stage in something like green bean casserole or a humble side dish.

12. Avocados

I absolutely love avocados, and the constantly growing sales numbers seem to suggest that other people are coming around. With the rise of vegetarianism and veganism, avocados have proven to be a great source of healthy fat and calories outside of meat.

There's nothing like fork-mashing a fresh avocado, adding some finely chopped tomato and your favorite spices for a homemade guacamole.

13. Green Onions

Green onions are a great topper for many dishes. If store-bought, keep them in their bag in your refrigerator with a little water covering the roots. They'll stay fresh for a long time, and keep their wonderful crispness. I like putting them on top of chilis and soups, personally.

14. Carrots

Just like cauliflower, carrots are extremely versatile. Depending on their preparation, they can be rich and savory, light and sweet, or fresh and vibrant. Many people over-boil their carrots, robbing them of their characteristic flavor, and it's a shame. Experiment a little, and find out how you like them!

15. Bok choy

Americans are finally coming around to what the Chinese have been onto for ages-- bok choy. It's a thick, stalked relative of napa cabbage, and it's super delicious. In my experience, it's a wonderful addition to stir fry, soup, and even on its own (the leaves, anyway) on sandwiches.

16. Apples

Apples are a great snack, and you've likely heard as much for most of your life. You were probably stuck with one of three varieties-- Red Delicious, Golden Delicious, and Granny Smith. Over its history (over 100 years, now), the Red Delicious as we know it has undergone a huge change, much of it in the last 30-40 years. It's been turned into a mockery of what it was, now thick-skinned and mushy, deep red to hide bruises and prevent preemptive spoilage. Demand is down in a big way, and with good reason.

A lot of new entries are gaining steam in the United States, most notably the Honeycrisp, Gala, and Fuji apples. Pick a few up soon.

You'll find a very different apple to the one you were likely to pick up before. Sweet, exceedingly crisp and fresh, wonderfully complex in some cases. These apples can be used for cooking, for pies and cakes, or applesauce-- anything you like. They're versatile and wonderful. There are far more varieties than the three I listed above, though-- the Rome apple, for example, is perfect for applesauce, with its rich, almost savory taste and exceedingly soft flesh. Experiment!

17. Oranges and related citrus

I love citrus. There are innumerable varieties, each with their own unique attributes and uses. There are, of course, the common sorts-- navel oranges, blood oranges, ruby red grapefruit, and so on. I'd like to draw attention to my favorite citrus fruit.

The Sumo Orange has been a work-in-progress in Japan for over 30 years, now. It's only been available for 3 years as of the publication date of this book, but it's garnering wide praise. Despite being what most would consider exceptionally ugly, it's being hailed as the most delicious orange ever, and I'm inclined to agree. It's exceedingly easy to peel, sweet, and clean. They're available from February to May in only certain stores (Whole Foods is where I get mine), being hand cultivated in California alone.

That particular example aside, citrus fruits are wonderful to keep around the house. They're a great source of vitamin C, something far too many people fall short on. I love using citrus to bring to life jellies, jams, and preserves (especially strawberry).

18. Lemons and limes

On the subject of citrus, lemons and limes are indispensable. While the lemon is much more commonly used for its tart flavor, limes have their place in any well stocked kitchen too.

While lemon juice can be applied most anywhere, lime juice works best in sweet things, or to balance out spice. Later in this book, you'll find a recipe for delicious Pad Thai which makes use of lime. In my opinion, it's the defining character of the finished dish, along with the crushed peanuts.

19. Bananas

Bananas, in addition to being a great snack, are a great source of potassium, absolute essential if you work out or have a physically demanding job. They're great at perking you up when you're tired and drained as well!

My favorite usage is in the pancake recipe I detail in Chapter 5.

20. Seasonal berries and fruit

If you're shopping at farmer's markets for your produce, chances are you'll be buying seasonally. It's important to know the harvest and sale seasons of to more common berries and fruits.

For example, blackberries are harvested and sold between May and October, while blueberries are only available fresh between May and August. On the flip side, grapefruit are available from December to April, as are most large citrus. Oranges are available year-round, thankfully!

Whatever your favorite fruit or berry is, be sure to learn when you can get them fresh. Don't worry if they're out of season, though-- some small chain grocers buy bulk from local suppliers and freeze for the off-season, and frozen is often just as good!

Stocking Your Pantry

In my opinion, there are two absolutely necessary things for any pantry, both from an economic and nutritional standpoint. First, dried beans, and almost any sort will do. Navy, kidney, black-- doesn't matter. So long as you have a ready supply of delicious protein and starch on tap, you'll be set.

The second is a reliable, stable grain. I prefer brown rice for this purpose, but most any rice (aside from the nutritionally deficient parboiled) will do the job. Buying rice and beans in bulk will ensure that even the hardest of times will pass right by you, as pairing the two will more often than not provide you with all the necessary proteins and carbohydrates for energy.

Aside from these two absolute essentials, you can also stock up on more "luxury" items like quinoa and chia. If you want an incredibly versatile and inexpensive alternative to beans, look to the lentil. It's packed with nutrition and protein, and is wonderfully delicious when prepared properly.

There are plenty of different grains and beans available, and you should buy small until you find something you know you like. At the end of this book, I provide a Cajun Red Beans & Rice recipe I'm sure you'll love.

Spices

The four basic spices are inexpensive, and you likely have them in your kitchen already-- salt, pepper, garlic powder, and onion powder. These are absolute necessities for cooking wholesome dinners at home. There a few other key items that, to me, make a well stocked spice cabinet.

Cumin is an all-too-often overlooked spice in English-speaking countries. It's extremely popular in Indian and South American cuisine, and has many beneficial effects such as aiding in digestion. It has a distinct, warm scent, and adds a wonderful richness to almost any dish. I really enjoy it in chilis and stews, but it's best to add it a bit at a time. In my experience, in periods of high cumin consumption, I've found myself losing quite a bit of weight, likely due to its positive effect on satiety, or the feeling of being full and satisfied.

Red pepper flakes can bring a lot of zing into an otherwise bland dish, and can go a long way in saving something that didn't quite come out the way you planned. In the same sense, cayenne is very useful, though its applications are far more diverse. If you go overboard with either, simply adding an acidic juice like lemon will neutralize much of the spice.

Allspice and lemon pepper are all more specialized spices, but are important in their own right. Allspice, especially when combined with cumin, is exceptional for roasting chicken. Lemon pepper flavors tilapia wonderfully, and in fact is wonderful on almost any seafood.

There are innumerable spices, and it's worth trying everything out, but these basics will get you started.

Chapter 3: Health Benefits

The average American consumes 2700 calories and 126 grams of sugar every day. The recommended daily allowances are 2000 and 25, respectively. Of course, the daily caloric needs are different for every person, but our current obesity epidemic (over 60% of Americans are overweight) displays the need for calorie restriction well enough.

But it's not just calorie restriction. Higher sugar intake, especially of processed and refined sugars, is linked heavily to weight gain. The advent of fast food restaurants and heavily processed food full of fats and sugars is largely to blame for the obesity epidemic, there can be no doubting that. A whole food, clean diet completely sidesteps the issues that plague most Americans and many around the world.

The USDA has a very basic recommendation for what an average dinner should consist of, and I'm in complete agreement. Half of your plate should be comprised of vegetables or fruit. The remaining quarters should be protein and grain.

Consider: a plate comprised of one cup cooked red beans, one cup brown rice, and 2 cups of Bird's Eye Normandy blend looks like this. 446 calories, 40 grams of protein, 4% of your sodium RDA, 8 grams of sugar, and 2 grams of fat.

If you eschew whole ingredients and get each component of the meal above from manufacturers (Blue Runner beans, Uncle Ben's rice, Del Monte mixed vegetables), here's what it looks like. 630 calories, 14 grams of sugar, a whopping 71% of your sodium, 5 grams of fat, and only 31 grams of protein. This is to say nothing of the preservatives and preparation issues.

The whole food preparation contains less calories, nearly half the sugar, less than half the fat, and just under one twentieth the sodium. I think the difference is clear.

This is a very simple example, but it's very illustrative. The simple act of paying more attention to the content of the food you buy has the potential to benefit you in huge ways. Even moreso if you ditch pre-prepared food entirely, working completely from whole ingredients. Research the companies you buy from, learn about their practices and business models, and understand where your food comes from. It couldn't be more important.

Chapter 4: Sourcing Your Ingredients

The biggest question raised when clean eating is brought up is a worthwhile one-- where do you get your ingredients? I'd like to show you how and where you can source the best ingredients for your meals.

The first important venue to mention is the age-old farmer's market. With the advent of large chain grocery stores, farmer's markets have become less and less common. But luckily for you, this also means that they price their goods competitively and strive to offer the best possible product to their customers. The average vendor at a farmer's market is likely to know that their customer-base is health-conscious and looking for clean, whole ingredients, and will provide.

Thumb through your local newspaper, especially in early Spring and late Summer, to find out about local markets and events. Learn about harvest schedules in your area to find out when you should be keeping an eye out for your favorite ingredients. You can feel good knowing that you've supported a local business, too!

The ability to talk to the people who grow the food for sale can do much to put your mind at ease about the path of your food from harvest to table, as well. Be sure to ask about anything that concerns you, whether it's the seed source or pesticide usage. You might learn quite a bit about the craft as well!

Speaking of, there's no better way to be sure of your food's origins than to simply grow it yourself. For most people, large scale growing is simply not a possibility, but everyone from apartment-dwellers and trailer-tenants to ranchers with plenty of land can grow *something*. Tomato plants can even be grown upside down, hanging in a window!

With a minimal investment, you can plant a few choice crops and tend them for a consistent source of delicious food. Tomatoes, as I said above, are a popular choice. Many people in the American South grow their own squash and peppers.

If you compost your food waste, you'll have a wonderful starting soil additive for most any crop. Be sure to read up on the requirements for each plant, including their preferred growing climate, soil necessities, tending, and pest control. Growing your own food is extremely rewarding, and can reduce your costs significantly!

Chapter 5: 25 Delicious Recipes for Every Meal

In this chapter, I'll give you 25 wonderful, simple recipes to get you started on your clean eating journey. I sometimes reference commonly pre-made ingredients (tortillas, pasta, etc), but these can be made easily enough at home. As with most recipes, they've been collected and changed over the years I've been cooking, and some have their roots in other recipes. Enjoy!

Breakfast

Pancakes

1.5 cups flour

1 cup milk mixed with 1 tablespoon apple cider vinegar

2 bananas

2 teaspoons baking powder

2 tablespoons corn starch

3 tablespoons sugar

2 teaspoons vanilla

1 pinch of salt

This recipe is great if you have an electric griddle, because you can dramatically shorten your cook time.

You're going to want to counter-ripen bananas until the peels are streaked brown and black. Definitely not rotten, but let them over-ripen a little. Mash them thoroughly in a large mixing bow, then adding the milk and vanilla. Combine the mixture, then place it aside.

Mix your dry ingredients, then pour the banana and milk mixture in. Stir until everything has incorporated to make a smooth batter. After oiling your griddle, grab a ¼ cup dry measure, spooning the mixture into it. Tilt the measure over the griddle, scooping the sides with the spoon, then smoothing out your pancake. When you start to see significant bubbling at the sides, flip with a thin-edged pancake turner. On an average griddle, you can cook 6-8 at a time. This recipe makes about a dozen of the best pancakes you'll ever have in my opinion, and you can easily add your favorite finely chopped fruit!

Morning Oats

½ cup steel cut oats

½ cup milk or yogurt

¼ cup fruit (your choice)

1 teaspoon vanilla

1 pinch of salt

1 tablespoon honey or maple syrup

1 tablespoon chia seeds (optional, but will make your oats thicker)

Combine all ingredients in a mason jar and mix well. Make sure to cap it tightly! Leave in the fridge overnight. Extremely simple recipe, and unbelievably delicious.

Cinnamon Rolls

1 cup milk

8 tablespoons butter

1 teaspoon salt

½ tablespoon of ground cinnamon

¼ cup of granulated sugar

Packet activated yeast

3 cups unbleached flour

Heat milk and 3 tablespoons of butter in your microwave until they melt, then let the mixture cool-- but not so long that it gets too thick. Pour this into your mixing bowl, add the yeast, then wait about 10 minutes. Next, a tablespoon of granulated sugar and a teaspoon of salt, stirring gently until thoroughly mixed.

Add your flour a bit at a time until it thickens and becomes sticky. Flour a cutting board, flipping and kneading the dough until it's a nice ball. Rinse your bowl, coat it with the oil of your choice and drop the dough back in, covering with cling wrap. You'll have to wait an hour or so before proceeding.

When your dough has risen properly, it's time to roll! On the cutting board you used earlier, roll the dough out to cover. Melt an additional 3 tablespoons of butter, then sprinkling on ¼ cup sugar and ½ or 1 tablespoon of cinnamon, depending on how much you like. Roll the dough up in a nice, tight spiral, then cut into rounds about 2 inches thick with your sharpest knife, careful to keep the sections intact. Brush with 2 more tablespoons of melted butter, cover with cling wrap, and place on top of the oven while you heat it to 350. Pop them in once your indicator beeps, and let them bake for about half an hour. If they're still a little soft, repeat in 5 minute increments.

Avocado Biscuits

Biscuits:

2 cups whole wheat flour

1 tablespoon baking powder

½ teaspoon baking soda

¾ teaspoon coarse salt

4 tablespoons unsalted butter

1 cup milk

1 tablespoon lemon juice

Preheat your oven to 450. Mix baking powder, flour, baking soda, and salt, then incorporating the butter with your hands until you have a thick mixture. Don't knead so long that the butter melts, you want to keep it at least semi-solid. Pour the milk in a quarter cup at a time, because you might not need the entire cup. If it seems too wet, you can add a little flour to thicken the mixture up, but expect it to be fairly sticky.

Knead the dough lightly on a floured surface, then breaking off enough to make a thick round of about an inch. Form in your hands, then place gently in an oiled baking dish or parchment paper covered pizza pan. Bake for about 15 minutes, making sure the tops look browned and somewhat crisp.

Avocado Mix:

2 large avocados

Onion powder

Garlic powder

Salt

Pepper

Red pepper flakes

Paprika

This recipe uses 2 avocado, but if you're making this for a large group, just use more avocados and adjust seasoning accordingly. This is a very 'to taste' recipe, so taste as you go! Simply fork-mash the avocados in a bowl, adding the listed seasonings as you like. When it's just right, place it aside in the fridge. Either cover or fill your finished biscuits for a great start to your day.

Big Bang Shake

This is my favorite quick morning recipe, and it couldn't be simpler.

Pour 1.5 cups of your favorite ground coffee into a 1 liter pitcher, then filling the rest with cold water. Using a silicon spatula or other long implement, stir thoroughly. Cover tightly, and place in the fridge to sit overnight.

In the morning, you'll have delicious cold-brew coffee. Drop a scoop of your favorite protein powder (I'm a huge fan of Sun Warrior's Warrior Blend) into your blender, then pouring the cold-brew coffee through a strainer (I prefer fine mesh tea strainers for this purpose). Mix, bottle, and go! Caffeine and protein are the ultimate morning starters, and this has plenty of both.

Lunch

Gargantuan Salad (makes 2)

Salad:

1 medium to large zucchini

1 medium to large yellow squash

1 cucumber

1 very large or 2 smaller carrots

1 tomato, diced

1 red bell pepper or ½ of both red and green depending on flavor preference

1 cup raw spinach per salad

1 avocado for topping (optional)

Shred carrot, zucchini, squash with a food processor or ajulienner. Thinly slice cucumber with knife or food processor. Lay ingredients on top of the bed of spinach. Dice tomato and bell pepper, place on top. Slice avocado and top. Drizzle dressing on top (below).

Dressing:

¼ cup chickpeas

1 tablespoon tahini

¼ to ½ cup water, depending on the thickness desired

¼ cup lemon juice

1-2 tablespoons soy sauce or tamari

1 tablespoon ground flaxseed (also known as flaxmeal)

1-2 cloves garlic

2 teaspoon minced ginger or ginger powder

black pepper to taste

Place all ingredients in a blender and blend until smooth. Set in fridge to chill and thicken. Add the rest of the water by teaspoon if it is too thick for your taste.

Summer Wraps

Traditional tortilla

Homemade refried beans

1 orange bell pepper, sliced and de-seeded

Spinach

Tomato, sliced into thin wedges

Spanish rice or wild rice

Avocado, either sliced thin or mashed

Salsa

This is a great, freshing mid-day lunch for light days. Simply heat your refried beans and rice, mixing thoroughly, then spreading onto a tortilla (if you're unfamiliar with making tortillas, there are innumerable guides available). Add the rest of your ingredients, rolling tightly, and dig in!

Baked Kale Chips

This is by far the most subjective recipe on this list, and it's almost impossible to quantify anything but the most basic aspects of making these chips.

First, you'll need two large bunches of kale. Cut the thick stems out, leaving only the leaves. The water in the stems will keep the kale from drying out correctly in the oven. Many people like them spicy, and therefore use cayenne and powdered garlic primarily. This recipe may take a few attempts before you get them the way you like them, but the basic prep and process is the same. Mix your oil and spices in a bowl, then evenly coating each of the leaves. Lay them out flat on whatever oven-safe dishes you have (pizza pans, baking sheets, cookie trays, doesn't matter) and bake for about 10 minutes at 350 degrees. You want them nice and crisp, but still green. If they go brown, you've left them on too long.

If you make a large batch like this once a week and store them in airtight bags, you'll always have a quick lunch snack if you're on the run.

Avocado Pasta

4 avocados, peeled and pitted

Splash of sherry cooking wine

1 tablespoon apple cider vinegar

2-4 cloves garlic, peeled and pressed

Salt, pepper, and onion powder to taste

Red pepper flakes-- ½ teaspoon or to taste

Splash to ½ cup milk

Combine all ingredients except the milk in your food processor. Gradually add milk until the sauce is as thick as you like it. Adjust seasoning and pour over pasta.

Hummus and Pita

Hummus:

1.5 cups cooked chickpeas

Few tablespoons to ¼ cup tahini

1-2 cloves garlic, pressed and/or minced

Teaspoon salt or to taste

Tablespoon lemon juice

2 tablespoons olive oil

2 tablespoons to ¼ cup water

Place chickpeas in processor, blend. Add tahini and garlic. Blend. Add lemon, salt, and olive oil. Blend. Add in water gradually until thickness is desired. To top: olives, roasted red pepper, artichoke, pine nuts.

Pita:

1 package active dry yeast

1 cup warm water

2 3/4 cup flour, divided and more for sprinkling

1 ½ tablespoon olive oil + 1 teaspoon

2 teaspoon salt

Whisk together warm water and 1 cup flour. Add yeast and stir gently. Let stand 15-20 minutes until foamy and bubbly.

Pour 1 ½ tablespoon olive oil, 1 ¾ cup flour, and salt into the foamy mixture. Stir together until the dough gets too thick, then gently mix by hand or with dough hook on a stand mixer. If dough sticks to side of the bowl, add flour a little at a time-- up to ¼ cup.

Knead dough until slightly springy and soft, about five minutes. Turn dough out onto a floured surface and form into a ball. Wipe inside of bowl with ¼ teaspoon olive oil, place doughball inside, and cover with plastic wrap or tin foil. Let rise 2 hours or until dough has doubled in size.

Remove dough and place back onto floured surface. Pat into a flat shape 1 inch thick. Cut into 8 pieces. Form each piece into a small round smooth ball, pulling dough from sides and tucking ends under the bottom. Sprinkle a little more flour onto workplace and on top of the dough and gently pat flat into a round disc about ¼ inch thick. Let rest for 5 minutes. Repeat with the other balls.

Brush a cast-iron skillet with remaining oil and place over medium-high heat. Lay the dough carefully into the skillet and cook until bread begins to get puffy and the bottom has brown spots and 'blisters', about 3 minutes. Flip, cook 2 mor3e minutes, and flip back onto original side for 30 seconds more. Stack cooked bread onto a plate and cool.

Dinner

Cajun Red Beans and Rice

2lbs uncooked red beans

Enough home-made vegetable broth, water, or a mix to cover the beans in a large crock pot and about an inch above; about 8-10 cups

1 bunch green onion, chopped

1 large yellow onion, either stripped or diced

4-6 cloves of garlic, minced

1 small green and 1 small red bell pepper, diced OR half of each of a larger size

1/4 cup fresh parsley, chopped finely

1 stalk celery, chopped finely (optional)

1 tablespoon liquid smoke

¼ cup burgundy cooking wine

2 whole bay leaves

3-4 tomatoes, juice included

1 tablespoon lemon juice

Cajun seasoning: 2teaspoon garlic powder, onion powder, paprika, cumin, oregano, red pepper flakes, salt, pepper, and cayenne; although you may want to only add half of a teaspoon cayenne if you don't like it too hot.

Combine water, wine, beans, liquid smoke, bay leaves, parsley and Cajun seasoning mix in a pot. If using a slow cooker, set to low for 8-10 hours or high for 4-6 hours. If using stovetop method, bring beans to a boil, set to medium low, add the above mentioned ingredients, and cover. Stir occasionally. If the beans look a bit dry, add more water ¼ cup at a time. Beans should be, after 2-3 hours of cooking, soft and will have made their own gravy. If desired, mash some of the beans with spoon or potato masher and mix. In the last hour of cooking, add the fresh ingredients- garlic, onion, celery, bell pepper, tomato and lemon juice. Serve over rice (2 cups uncooked rice will cover almost the whole pot; cook separately).

Hearty Home Stew

2 large russet potatoes, chopped into smaller chunks

2 large or 3 medium carrots, sliced into rounds

1 red bell pepper, diced

1 green bell pepper, diced

2 tomatoes, diced

2 cups spinach or 1 bunch kale, chopped

2 bags white pearl onions, peeled

6 cloves garlic, pressed and minced

2 cobs' worth of corn, cooked and kernels cut from the cob

1 lb green beans

Cumin

Salt

Pepper

Cayenne to taste

Garlic and onion powder

4 cups vegetable broth

Combine broth and potatoes in a large pot. Bring to a boil and cook the potatoes until they are very, very soft, even falling apart. This is what will make your stew thick. Add all other ingredients and more broth, if necessary. Cook about 3 hours covered on medium-low.

Summer Chili

1 medium zucchini

1 medium squash

2 cobs' worth corn, cooked and kernels cut away from cob

2 large tomatoes, diced

2 28oz jars tomato sauce

1/2lb chili beans

1/2lb red beans

4-6 cups vegetable broth

1 red bell pepper and 1 green bell pepper, diced

1 large onion, stripped

3 cloves garlic, minced

1lb portabella mushrooms, sliced

3 teaspoons chili powder

2 teaspoons salt

1 teaspoon cumin

2 teaspoons pepper

1teaspoon garlic and onion powder

Combine broth and beans (using enough broth to cover the beans and an additional half-inch) and cook for about 2 hours on medium-low heat. Add all other ingredients and cook for another few hours, adjusting seasonings and stirring frequently. Serve with favorite cheese and green onions on top.

Fried Rice

2 cups uncooked rice, prepared and stored overnight

1 head broccoli, chopped into tiny trees

2 cups peas

1 onion, diced

1 red and 1 green bell pepper (or half of each), diced

¼ cup rice vinegar

¼ cup tamari or soy sauce

2 teaspoons sriracha sauce

3 teaspoons Chinese Five Spice mix

2 tablespoon oil, divided

Mix rice vinegar, tamari/soy, and rooster sauce together in a small cup and set aside. In a large frying pan or wok, heat 1 tablespoon oil and toss in the broccoli, onion, garlic, and bell peppers and cook about 5 minutes over medium-high heat. Add the peas in the last minute or two of cooking. Toss on the five spice seasoning, mix well, and transfer the vegetables into a bowl for now. Heat the last tablespoon oil, then cook the rice. Pour the vinegar/soy sauce mixture on top of the rice, adding more by the teaspoon each if it isn't coated enough. Cook rice about five minutes, stirring often so it doesn't burn, then add in the vegetables. Mix well, cook another minute or two, and serve. Add-ins include chicken, pork, or tofu.

Pad Thai

4oz noodle of choice-- Udon or fettuccine-style rice noodle works best

2-4 tablespoons tamarind paste

¼ cup peanut or sesame oil

¼ cup soy sauce or tamari

¼ cup honey

2 tablespoons rice vinegar

½ teaspoon red pepper flakes or to taste

1 stalk green onions, chopped

1 garlic clove, minced

2 eggs

4 cups shredded napa cabbage (or whichever you can find)

1lb chicken, shrimp, or pressed tofu

Garnish:

1 cup mung bean sprouts

½ cup peanuts, roasted and crushed finely

1-2 limes, quartered

Cook noodles according to directions (it will be different between udon and rice noodle). Drain and toss with 1 tablespoon oil and set aside.

Mix together the honey, tamarind paste, vinegar, and soy or tamari sauce in a small saucepan and heat over low. Stir in the red pepper flakes and set aside. In a large skillet or wok, add the remaining oil over medium-high. Add the green onions and garlic and cook for about a minute. Add in the eggs and allow to cook for about 30-seconds before scrambling. Add in the cabbage and cook until cabbage is wilted. Here, you can add diced chicken breast or pressed tofu. Cook thoroughly. When the chicken is white or the tofu begins to brown, add both noodles and sauce and cook until noodles are warmed through. When serving, place mung beans on top, sprinkle the crushed roasted peanut on top, and squeeze the lime wedges.

Buffalo Chicken Sandwich and Potato Wedges

Buffalo sauce is a lot easier to make at home than people think. I like to use Frank's cayenne sauce as a base. Since it only really contains simple ingredients (aged peppers, vinegar, water, salt, garlic powder), there's no need to question the fitness for any dish it's added to.

1 cup Frank's hot saucepan

2 tablespoons oil (your choice, canola works best for me)

2 tablespoons all purpose flour

1 tablespoon vinegar (white or apple cider, either is fine)

¼ cup warm water

Just drop the oil in a saucepan on medium heat, pour your flour in and stir til it browns up. Add in half of your hot sauce, stir until mixed, then add the rest of your ingredients. When it's all together and mixed, take it off of the heat and place aside. You just made what I consider the most delicious buffalo sauce around, using the same base as the guy who invented it. It's wonderfully thick and sticks well to whatever you coat in it. Doesn't get better than that.

As for the chicken, all you really need to do is get as many deboned, skinless chicken breasts as you intend to eat, drop them in a well oiled slow cooker, add your delicious sauce, and cook for about 6 hours. When that's all done, shred with a fork, add to your favorite bun or bread, and dig in.

But not before you have your fries!

2 very large potatoes or 3-4 medium ones

2 tablespoons corn starch

2 tablespoons coconut oil in liquid form

1-2 teaspoons salt

1-2 teaspoons pepper

2 teaspoons paprika

1 teaspoon cumin

2 teaspoon dried parsley

½ teaspoon cayenne

Cut the large potatoes into eights (less or more, depending on how thick you like them, though I'd suggest eights for an even cook), then place them into a gallon bag with the corn starch and liquid coconut oil. Shake to coat, then dropping the spices in and doing the same.

On a large pizza pan, place some parchment paper and oil it. Position the fries so that none are touching if possible, then cook at 450 for 25 minutes on each side. Make sure you keep an eye on them during the second cycle to ensure that they don't burn!

Tilapia

1 large tilapia fillet

½ stripped onion

1 stripped bell pepper

3 tablespoons lemon juice

2 cloves minced garlic

Lemon pepper to taste

This is a pretty simple recipe, but it's always a big hit. Strip your onion and bell pepper, making a bed in a large broiler pan. Lay the tilapia fillet atop the bed, then coating with the lemon juice and lemon pepper. Mince the garlic, placing half atop the fillet and sprinkling the rest across the bed.

Broil for 5-7 minutes on each side, turning once. When you pull it out, let it stand for a few minutes and serve, taking some of the vegetable bed with you as you do. Works well on its own or with lemon rice on the side!

Savory Tempeh Sandwiches

1 8oz package Westsoy tempeh (or your preferred brand)

2 tablespoons butter

2 tablespoons burgundy red cooking wine

1 tablespoon soy sauce or tamari (I prefer tamari for its lower sodium)

½ teaspoon garlic powder

½ teaspoon onion powder

This is a relatively quick, light dinner for those nights when you just don't have time for a big meal. If you're not familiar with tempeh, get acquainted. Tempeh originated in Indonesia, and it's absolutely delicious. It's a fermented soy product, and comes in a packed, solid rectangular piece.

Add your spices, oil, and wine to the pan. Cut your tempeh into strips, then frying on either side on medium-high heat for about 5 minutes, or until browned. Serve on toasted bread with your favorite sandwich fixings. Because of the rich, savory character of this dish, I recommend pairing it with a light cheese, spinach, and a spicy tomato sauce. Kale chips are great on the side!

Stuffed Bell peppers

6 bell peppers (red/green/yellow, no orange) sliced lengthways in half

1 onion, diced fine

1 cup rice, cooked in vegetable or chicken broth

2 cloves garlic, minced

1/2 cup tomato sauce

1 teaspoon salt

1 lb ground turkey (optional)

teaspoon chili powder

1lb cheddar cheese (plus mozzarella to top if desired)

Sauté onion and garlic in a bit of oil until fragrant. Add the ground turkey and cook thoroughly. In a large mixing bowl, mix the rice, seasonings, cheese and tomato sauce. Add in the turkey mixture. Mix well and scoop into the halved and cleaned bell peppers. Top with more cheese if desired and cooked covered for 30 minutes covered and another 10 uncovered or until peppers are tender.

Jambalaya

3 cups uncooked rice

1 tablespoon tomato paste

2 diced tomatoes

1 medium onion, diced

1 bunch of green onions, diced

2-4 cloves garlic, minced

1 green and 1 red bell pepper, diced

1 bunch fresh parsley, chopped fine

1 stalk celery, chopped

7.5 cups vegetable or chicken broth

teaspoon garlic and onion powder

cayenne powder, to taste

red pepper flakes, to taste

½ teaspoon cumin

1 teaspoon paprika

Teaspoon liquid smoke

Salt and pepper, to taste

1lb shredded chicken or cubed firm tofu

If you are using shredded chicken, it's best to marinate it overnight in a spice blend. If you are using tofu, read down to the end.

In a very large pot, combine all ingredients (unless you're using tofu; leave that out). Add a tablespoon of butter, bring to a boil, then simmer covered for about an hour or until the rice looks fluffy and done. This can also be cooked in your rice cooker-- just follow the water requirements for 3 cups of rice instead.

If using tofu, prepare it at the end. Roll it in a few shakes of hot sauce, liquid smoke, tamari or soy sauce, and some garlic and onion powder. Fry it in a skillet until all the liquid is absorbed and the tofu has taken on that wonderful smoky-orange look. Add to the jambalaya after it's finished cooking. This keeps as leftovers just as well as the chicken.

Desserts

Chia pudding

¼ cup chia seeds

1 cup milk of choice

¼ teaspoon vanilla extract

Pinch salt

1 tablespoon honey or other sugar

Fruit, nut, or granola to top

Combine all ingredients (except granola and nut, if using) in either a mason jar or large cup, then placing in the refrigerator for at least an hour. Sprinkle on any desired toppings when you bring it out.

Rice pudding

2 cups cooked rice

1 cup milk of choice (add more if it's too thick for you)

¼ cup sugar (or more-- check sweetness!)

1-2 teaspoon cinnamon

1 teaspoon cinnamon

One drop almond emulsion (optional, but amazing)

Combine all ingredients into a pot. Bring to a boil and let simmer on medium-low for 20-30 minutes, stirring occasionally. The pudding will still appear a bit thin, but this is fine. Turn the heat off and let the pudding sit for 10-20 minutes. Taste, add more sweetener if desired, and add another splash or two of milk if the consistency is too thick.

Almond Sugar Cookies

1 ½ cups flour

¼ teaspoon salt

¼ teaspoon baking soda

⅛ teaspoon cinnamon (optional)

2 Tablespoons melted coconut oil

1 ¼ teaspoons vanilla extract

¼ teaspoon almond extract or two drops almond emulsion (I prefer this for its stronger, more accurate taste)

¼ cup pure maple syrup or raw cane sugar

Almond slivers for topping (optional)

Preheat oven to 325F while you prepare the cookies. Mix together the dry ingredients. In another bowl, melt the coconut oil in the microwave and add the sweetener, vanilla and almond extracts. Mix together, then combine with the dry ingredients. You may need to play around a little-- Sometimes you may need more coconut oil or more flour. You want it to be a little sticky, but not so wet that it won't form into the shape you want it to. Add more sugar if you need to. Line your baking sheet with parchment paper or spray it down and scoop out your cookies using a regular eating teaspoon. You should get about 15 cookies give or take depending on the size.

Once they are pressed and flattened into the desired shape, you can place the almond slivers on top however you like. Make sure to press them in a little. Bake for 15-18 minutes, or until golden brown. Remove and let cool for 10 minutes before serving.

Yogurt Parfait

1 container of vanilla yogurt or 1/2 cup

¼ cup fruit of choice (Strawberries and blueberries work well here-- use both if you like!)

Granola and/or whipped cream, to top

Whipped cream:

1 can coconut milk, sat in the fridge for at least a day undisturbed

1-2 teaspoon powdered sugar

½ teaspoon vanilla

In your desired cup or small bowl, layer ¼ cup yogurt, the berries, more yogurt, and top with the whipped cream and granola.

For an easy, lighter whipped cream, gently take out that can of coconut milk, turn it upside down, and open the can. Try to disturb it as little as possible. Pour off the clear water and use it later for a smoothie or just drink it straight like I do. There should be a solid white chunk in the bottom of the can-- this is the gold you're looking for. Scoop that into a mixing bowl, add the sugar and vanilla, and beat on medium speed for 3-5 minutes until soft peaks form. If it seems a bit flat, add some solid coconut oil and whip some more.

Applesauce and Ice Cream

5lbs apples: Try to get a mix of at least Granny smith and Honeycrisp apples, but having some golden delicious apples in there will sweeten the deal even more.

½-1 cup sugar, depending on preference (I use a different amount each time depending on the way the apples turned out)

1-2 cups water (depending on consistency preference)

2-4 teaspoon cinnamon

Spritz lemon juice (optional)

Peel, core, and chop the apples up into little pieces. They don't have to be minced, but keep the pieces small enough to cook through properly. Toss them in a slow cooker (or a pot if you don't have one, but seriously, get one) with the sugar, cinnamon, and water (random tip: for more apple-y applesauce, use apple cider or juice instead of water). Using the high setting on your crock pot, for 4 hours, or on medium heat, covered in a pot until apples are soft enough to be mashed easily. Use a potato masher or your blender to blend the applesauce. If you prefer it chunky, I recommend the potato masher, but you can also just set aside some of the chunks and mix them in once you've blended, too. For an especially smooth sauce, use Rome apples.

Conclusion

Clean eating isn't an all-or-nothing proposition. Even making a few substitutions in your usual food fare can have a substantial effect on your health. I can't tell you to never buy processed food, only that when you do, knowing its origins and ingredients is absolutely essential to your well-being.

I hope this book has helped you to understand just what clean eating is, and the many ways in which it can benefit you. Armed with this knowledge, you're ready to begin. In this case as in all others, the destination is not what is important-- it's the journey. Making the essential lifestyle change of being aware of what you consume and choosing wisely can lead to great things, including weight loss and improved general health.

If you follow the guidelines outlined in this book, your body will be fueled properly for anything you ask of it, from exercise to increased productivity at work. When you eat well, the results speak for themselves.

I also hope you enjoy the recipes I've given you here. They include plenty of personal recipes, and while some of them take their inspiration from many other cooks and recipes old and new (as all recipes do), they're presented as I personally make them. Don't be afraid to experiment and change them yourself, turning them into your ideal dishes if they aren't already. That's what cooking is really about-- a march toward perfection for each person through building on what has worked for others.

Hope you've enjoyed this book, if so, please take a moment to leave a review. Also don't forget to check our my other books on the Kindle store listed below.

Thank you for reading.

K.A. DeWolf

Check Out My Other Books:

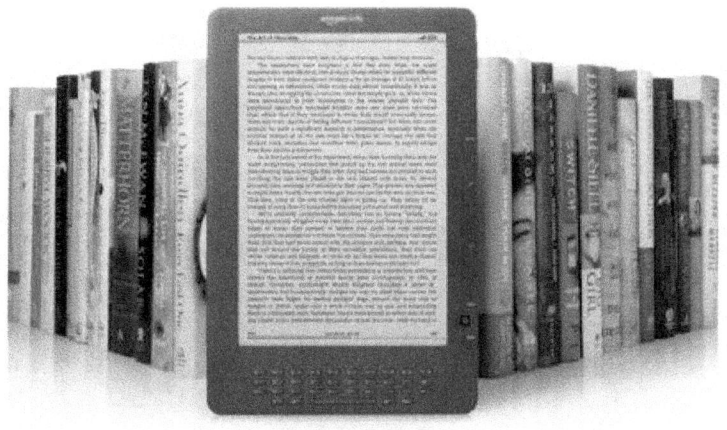

Memory Improvement:: 25 Powerful Ways to Improve Your Memory in 30 Days

Bullying: Stop Bullying; Effective Ways To Overcome Bullying In School Permanently: Modern Day Approach To Prevent Bullying Once And For All

Bootstrapping Entrepreneur: 100 Free Online Tools for Startups and First-Time Entrepreneurs: Small Business Tools For Entrepreneur Startup, Small Business Ideas, Online Tools for Business

Learn How to Use a Computer: 50 Tips and Suggestions to Help You Get the Most Out of Your Computer

Creative Thinking: What Top Creative People From Around The World Can Teach Us

Dog Sense: Top Lessons in Learning Dog Behavior and Understanding Your Dog

Clean Eating: The Amazing Way to Eat Healthy and Lose Weight (Includes 25 Recipes) – Avoid Processed Food and Reset Your Body's Natural Balance

FREE Kindle Books and New Kindle Book Announcements!

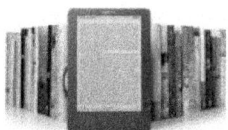

Join our exclusive readers club and receive notification when our books are FREE on Kindle Store for limited time. Also be the first to know about exciting new titles that are published every month for only $0.99.

*** We hate spam and never share your email with anyone ***

JOIN NOW!

www.ingramcontent.com/pod-product-compliance
Lightning Source LLC
Chambersburg PA
CBHW070827290526
45795CB00002B/862